Made in the USA
Las Vegas, NV
26 March 2021

20203895R00070